This reference book₁ awareness of Lyme Disease. The objectives of the reference booklet include that: (1) you understand the disease and how to prevent contracting it; (2) you know when and why to seek medical attention promptly; (3) you understand the consequences of untreated Lyme Disease, impacting your productivity and wasteful insurance spending; and (4) you seek skilled medical care if you might already have contracted Lyme Disease.

A glossary and phonetic pronunciation guide on the inside covers will aid your understanding of this material. Please feel free to share your reference resource with others. Understanding the risks of contracting Lyme Disease and the value of preventive measures will be your **best** protection.

Lyme Disease is a bacterial infection. It is transmitted to humans and other animals by the bite of an **infected**, hard-shelled deer tick. Not all deer ticks are infected with this bacteria. The percentage of infected ticks varies from neighborhood to neighborhood. If left untreated, a persistent bacterial infection results. Over time, Lyme Disease is characterized by several stages and sets of symptoms. If you live where Lyme Disease is widespread and occurs on a continuing basis (endemic area), understanding how to prevent getting Lyme Disease is your **best** protection. This reference booklet will educate you and your family about Lyme Disease.

What is Lyme Disease?

Lyme Disease is transmitted through the bite of an **infected** tick. The potentially serious bacterial infection exhibits numerous clinical symptoms and signs. Antibiotic drugs are used to treat all stages of Lyme Disease. Untreated, Lyme Disease may progress through several stages, most commonly affecting the skin, heart, nervous system, or joints. Less frequently, Lyme Disease affects other parts of the body, including the eyes, ears, liver, kidneys, and lungs.

In the earliest stages of the disease, antibiotic drugs are generally considered curative. Lyme Disease can range in severity from rather mild flu-like symptoms and rashes to much more serious consequences. If untreated during early stages,

Lyme Disease may become chronic and long-term, marked by relapses, remissions, and the need for retreatment. Without treatment, late Lyme Disease may result in obvious impairment and disability.

Speaking about Lyme Disease in the 1980s, Dr. Russell C. Johnson (U MN) said, "If it weren't for AIDS, it would be the Number One **new** disease facing us today." By 1989, the Centers for Disease Control (CDC) had counted 22,570 persons meeting strict criteria for Lyme Disease in the US. Some physicians and health department officials estimate that the actual number of Lyme Disease cases may be four to ten times higher than the CDC surveillance number.

Is Lyme Disease New?

In the US, the name Lyme Disease was coined in the mid-1970s describing an unusual clustering of juvenile rheumatoid arthritis-like cases in a few coastal towns near Lyme, CT. A peculiar rash often preceded the joint problems in about one-half of the children. This rash was quite similar to erythema chronicum migrans (ECM) seen in Europe. ECM was first described in the European literature in 1909. In 1969 the first US case of ECM was reported in a Wisconsin grouse-hunting physician. In museum specimens of small ticks collected on Long Island, NY in the 1940s, tick midgut contents were examined by DNA fingerprinting. Still present in the tick midgut were remains of *Borrelia burgdorferi*, the bacteria that causes Lyme Disease. *Borreliae* are corkscrew-shaped bacteria, classified as spirochetes.

During the last fifteen years, many physicians, laboratories, and field workers contributed to our current understanding of Lyme Disease. Migrating birds are believed to have transported infected ticks across the ocean from Europe more than 50 years ago. Through the behaviors of ground-feeding birds, field mice, and deer, Lyme Disease in the US now appears in wooded areas, open fields, coastal woodlands, nature preserves, and reclaimed agricultural lands. Many of these are adjacent to suburban neighborhoods with increasing frequency. Wherever the deer population is growing under protectionist policy moving closer to human habitats, conditions are favorable for the growth of Lyme Disease. Following the introduction of infected ticks, Lyme Disease begins to appear in humans and domestic pets.

Where Is Lyme Disease?

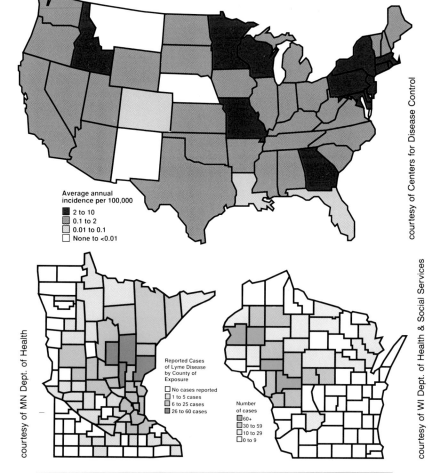

courtesy of Centers for Disease Control

courtesy of WI Dept. of Health & Social Services

courtesy of MN Dept. of Health

PREVALENCE OF LYME DISEASE CASES BY STATE IN THE U.S. 1988-1989.

Prior to 1991, each state used its own case definition of Lyme Disease so direct comparisons between states are not appropriate (see chart on page 21). Color code refers to incidences of reported cases per 100,000 during 1988-89.

Average annual
incidence per 100,000

- 2 to 10
- 0.1 to 2
- 0.01 to 0.1
- None to <0.01

Reported Cases
of Lyme Disease
by County of
Exposure

- No cases reported
- 1 to 5 cases
- 6 to 25 cases
- 26 to 60 cases

Number
of cases

- 60+
- 30 to 59
- 10 to 29
- 0 to 9

CUMULATIVE PREVALENCE OF LYME DISEASE IN MINNESOTA 1982-1990

Since 1982, Minnesota has reported 688 cases of Lyme Disease to the CDC, shown above by county of residence. The majority of cases occur in northeastern quadrant of MN, especially along the St. Croix River Valley.

CUMULATIVE PREVALENCE OF LYME DISEASE IN WISCONSIN 1980-1988

Since 1980, Wisconsin has reported 2428 cases of Lyme Disease to the CDC, shown by county of residence. The majority of cases occur in the northwestern quadrant of WI, but the disease is spreading slowly to the east and south.

Where is Lyme Disease?

Eight states in the northeastern and north central United States are considered endemic for Lyme Disease by the Centers for Disease Control. Endemic means that the disease is widespread and occurring on a continuing basis. In the Midwest, Minnesota and Wisconsin report many cases of Lyme Disease each year. In the Northeast, Connecticut, Rhode Island, New Jersey, Massachusetts, New York, and Pennsylvania are endemic areas.

However, Lyme Disease is not restricted to these eight states. Parts of California, Oregon, Texas, Louisiana, Florida, and Georgia report increasing problems with Lyme Disease. In fact, Lyme Disease has been identified in Europe, Asia, Africa, Canada, Central America, and Australia. Migratory birds appear to be responsible for the spread of infected ticks around the globe. Understanding where Lyme Disease is found and how to protect yourself is a must when travelling or vacationing.

The Tick Vector

Very small ticks belonging to the *Ixodes* family are the primary carriers of Lyme Disease. Varying percentages of these ticks are infected with the *Borrelia* bacteria. In most of the US, the deer tick or bear tick (*Ixodes dammini*) is responsible for disease transmission. In the western US states, the small black-legged tick (*Ixodes pacificus*) carries the Lyme bacteria. In Europe the most frequently infected tick species is the sheep tick (*Ixodes ricinus*). This tick occurs throughout southern Scandinavia, the British Isles, central Europe, France, Spain, Portugal, northern Italy, the Balkan countries, and the European regions of the USSR. In Asia, other small hard-bodied ticks (*Ixodes persulcatus*) are the predominant vector, or carrier of Lyme Disease.

Ixodes ticks generally progress through a two-year life cycle. In late summer and fall, the female receives a final blood meal, often from a deer, and then mates. Following copulation, the female drops to the ground, where she overwinters. In the spring the adult female lays eggs on the underside of brush or dried leaves. During July and August the eggs hatch, emerging as six-legged larvae. Passage of the bacterial infection from mother to eggs is inefficient, occurring about 1% of the time. Thus, most larvae will not be infected.

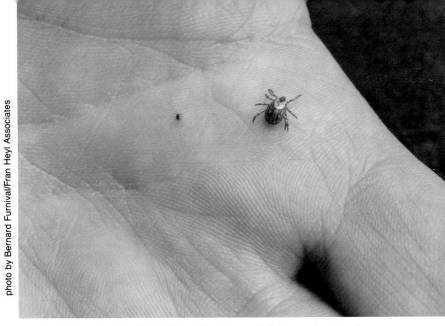

Female adult American dog tick (right) and deer tick nymph (left) on palm of man's hand. Deer tick nymph is responsible for 80% of human cases of Lyme Disease.

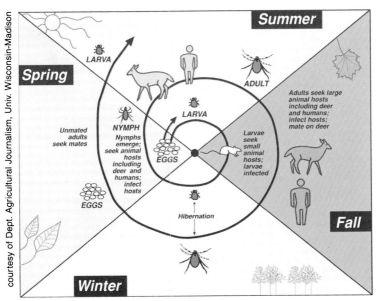

Summer

Spring

LARVA

ADULT

Adults seek large animal hosts including deer and humans; infect hosts; mate on deer

LARVA

Unmated adults seek mates

NYMPH
Nymphs emerge; seek animal hosts including deer and humans; infect hosts

Larvae seek small animal hosts; larvae infected

EGGS

EGGS

Hibernation

Fall

Winter

TWO-YEAR LIFE CYCLE OF THE DEER TICK

During each development stage, the larva, nymph, or adult tick needs one blood meal.

5

Larval stage ticks are often called "seed" ticks, sometimes resembling moving dust. Because of their exceedingly small size, the early habitat of larvae is among the forest, field, or lawn debris. The first blood meal of the larvae is usually taken from animals close to the ground, or from animals lying on the ground close to hatching sites. Larval ticks typically become infected by feeding on **infected** field mice. In the US, the white-footed field mouse is the primary reservoir for harboring *Borrelia* spirochetes. In turn, small ticks which become infected pass on the bacteria to larger hosts. To a lesser degree, other small mammals such as meadow voles, chipmunks, and rabbits may carry *Borreliae.*

Following a blood meal, larvae molt and mature. The following spring, larger eight-legged nymphal ticks emerge. Nymphs are visible, being about the size of poppy seeds or very small freckles. Nymphs may continue feeding activity throughout the summer and fall. Nymphs seek (quest) a host blood meal from the tips of vegetation, generally grasses ranging in height from a few inches to a foot or more. A potential host's body heat is detected by sensory organs on the tick's front legs. Once the ground has some snow cover, nymphs remain dormant during the late fall and winter. It is the **infected** nymphal form of the tick which transmits 80% of human cases of Lyme Disease, probably because it easily escapes detection. A feeding session lasts 3-5 days, and the engorged tick drops off, often unnoticed.

If unfed, the nymph will continue questing the following spring. Once fed, the nymph will molt into the adult tick in the summer. The adult female will require one more blood meal before mating and laying eggs. The adult form is about the size of the head of a pin, although it is too small to be felt crawling or biting. About 20% of human Lyme Disease is contracted from **infected** adult ticks.

It usually takes two years to complete this three-stage life cycle (larva, nymph, adult). More than 60% of the tick bites occur during June, July, and August. Fewer tick bites are reported during the spring and fall seasons, and just under 10% occur from December through February. Infected larval, nymphal, and adult forms of the tick are all capable of transmitting Lyme Disease to humans.

The female *Ixodes* tick is ideally designed for prolonged feeding, very often hidden from view. Feeding ticks usually seek out warm, moist skin folds. Using a serrated thrusting claw, the tick digs deep into the skin to locate a capillary, cementing its "mouthparts" in place. The tick also injects several substances to protect the feeding site. Anticoagulants maintain blood flow and immunosuppressants reduce localized reactions against contact with the tick. Laboratory animal studies suggest that at least 12-24 hours of feeding are needed before infected ticks begin to pass bacteria into the host's bloodstream. Daily body checks for attached ticks greatly reduce your chances of becoming infected with the *Borrelia* spirochete.

It is not known whether the tick's midgut colonies of spirochetes are regurgitated into the host during feeding. Spirochetes may migrate into the salivary gland of feeding ticks and then be passed to the host. Certainly, care must be taken when removing a feeding tick to avoid expelling tick contents into the host (see **Removal of the Tick**).

What Causes Lyme Disease?

Corkscrew-shaped bacteria called *Borrelia burgdorferi* are transmitted to the human bloodstream through the **prolonged** feeding of infected Ixodes ticks. Not every tick is infected with *Borreliae*. It is impossible to identify an infected tick without a laboratory examination. Infectivity rates in endemic regions vary from just a few per cent to more than 70% in the "hottest spots".

Borrelia burgdorferi belong to a group of bacteria called spirochetes. Comparison of *Borreliae* from infected *Ixodes* ticks in various parts of the world suggest only minor differences. Initially, scientists thought different strains might produce distinct clinical forms of Lyme Disease. For example, did the US have a higher proportion of arthritic complications compared to Europe? As physicians on both sides of the Atlantic looked for neurological (nervous system) manifestations, or different skin diseases, or cardiac involvement, American and European Lyme Disease appeared more similar than first thought.

Only *Borrelia burgdorferi* appears to cause Lyme Disease in humans and other animals. Recently, "Lyme borreliosis" is gaining acceptance to describe the infection caused by *Borrelia burgdorferi*. Other types of spirochetes are responsible for other human diseases. Spirochetal diseases are characterized by involvement of several organ and tissue systems, appearing to progress through several stages over prolonged periods of time. Syphilis, for example, is caused by the spirochete *Treponema pallidum.*

Spirochetal diseases, like syphilis or Lyme Disease, often begin with a skin abnormality. Without treatment, the skin clears up only to be replaced by other problems which appear unrelated. Lyme borreliosis is a multi-system, multi-phase disorder characterized by disease stages. These stages may be separated by several days to several months, or the stages may overlap. A particular stage may even be absent or so mild as to escape notice. Spirochetes like *Borrelia burgdorferi* are difficult to grow and study in culture outside the host. However, in the human host, the bacteria persist and multiply for years.

It is unclear how Lyme Disease becomes chronic and long-term. The mechanism underlying the chronic manifestations of Lyme Disease is unknown. Some believe that living *Borreliae* maintain the disease, while others feel that *Borreliae* trigger self-sustaining autoimmune responses directed against the self. Or, it may be a combination of both processes. *Borreliae* do travel to remote sites in the body via the bloodstream (dissemination of the disease). In these remote sites, the bacteria can persist for a very long time.

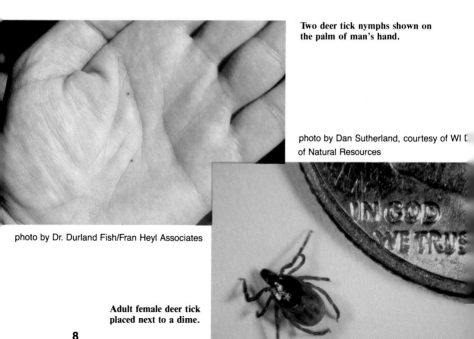

Two deer tick nymphs shown on the palm of man's hand.

photo by Dan Sutherland, courtesy of WI [of Natural Resources

photo by Dr. Durland Fish/Fran Heyl Associates

Adult female deer tick placed next to a dime.

Another feature of spirochetal diseases also helps promote the success of the infection. Like other spirochetes, *Borrelia burgdorferi* disguises or changes its appearance. The technical name for this maneuver is antigenic variation. Antigen describes a substance, an organism, or part of an organism, which appears foreign to your immune system. Antigens cause the release and production of antibodies. Generally, the body recognizes *Borreliae* as foreign by mounting an immune response. Bound antigen-antibody complexes are removed from the body. However, any remaining *Borreliae* may redisguise itself to avoid recognition by the immune system.

In addition to antigenic variation, *Borreliae*, like other spirochetes, reproduce much more slowly. *Borreliae* are able to undergo prolonged periods of latency (inactivity). Antibiotic drugs are directed at bacteria which are undergoing cell division. This makes *Borreliae* less vulnerable to antibiotic drugs than more rapidly-dividing bacteria.

Borreliae are also able to penetrate tissues such as brain, muscle sheaths, or joint fluids. In these tissues, direct blood contact is infrequent, thereby escaping many immune-mediated defenses (antibodies) or contact with circulating antibiotic drugs. Thus, long-term chronic Lyme borreliosis is more difficult to eradicate than most bacterial infections.

Early Signs and Symptoms of Lyme Disease

Following the bite of an infected deer tick, it is estimated that 50-70% of adults, and about 50% of children, will develop a characteristic rash at the bite site. The term "rash" is used in its broadest sense to define a change in the appearance of the skin, not necessarily the presence of broken skin, bumps, or blisters. Erythema migrans (EM) most typically appears between 3 and 30 days after the bite. EM consists of an expanding redness which surrounds the bite. As the redness grows in size, the center of the rash may clear and appear normal. This pattern is referred to as a bull's-eye rash.

EM may take forms other than the bull's-eye pattern. It may look like a red blotch, or develop into a festered sore. EM is most often rounded, but can appear in a variety of different shapes. EM may be flat or raised; it may burn, or itch, or even feel quite normal. In a few cases, EM may develop at several other sites, remote from the bite area. Or a series of red rings may encircle one another, resembling a tree-ring appearance (annular rash). Whatever shape or appearance the rash may take, it may remain small in size and disappear quickly, or it may grow over a period of weeks up to ten inches in diameter. It is impossible to describe all EM rashes simply in a few words. Any unusual appearance of the skin, especially in summer months, should prompt you to seek medical attention.

The change in the appearance of the skin at the bite site is due to the presence of the spirochetes in the skin. Culturing spirochetes from the red margins of the rash has become more successful in recent years. This method is seldom used for diagnosis. Likely places for the tick bite site, and hence, the EM to appear are on the thighs, in the groin, in moist skin folds, the underarms, neck, or scalp. For most, the rash usually disappears without treatment, within a few weeks. The rash should not be ignored.

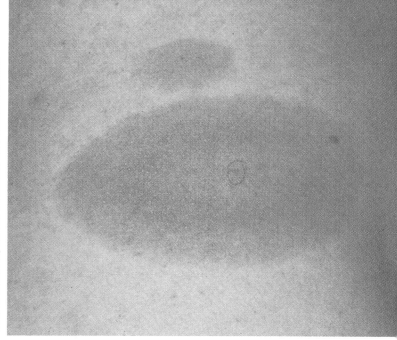

courtesy of Dept. Agricultural Journalism, Univ. Wisconsin-Madison

Characteristic bull's-eye rash on the back.

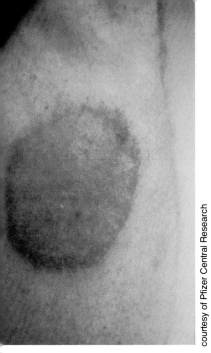

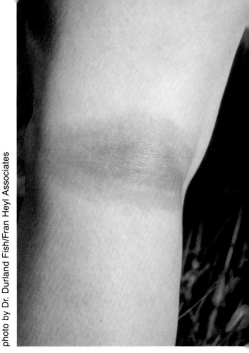

courtesy of Pfizer Central Research

photo by Dr. Durland Fish/Fran Heyl Associates

**thema migrans (EM) appearing as a red
on man's leg.**

**Erythema migrans (EM) appearing as a red
splotch behind woman's knee.**

The majority of patients developing EM also experience a variety of flu-like symptoms (constitutional symptoms). These would include headache, stiff neck, muscle aches and pains, conjunctivitis ("pink eye"), fever, chills, sore throat, fatigue, swollen lymph nodes, and general malaise. Like EM itself, the constitutional symptoms fade without treatment. Among the 20-40% of cases in which EM does not develop or is not noticed, similar nondescript symptoms may appear and disappear within a few days.

Early localized Lyme Disease had been called Stage 1. In the early disease, spirochetes are only found in the skin near the bite site and in the bloodstream. Early localized disease generally lasts a few days to a few weeks. If no treatment is given, about 80% of early Lyme Disease patients will progress to later disease stages. In its chronic stage, the disease is more severe and more difficult to treat. In the other 20% not receiving early treatment, the disease appears to be self-limiting. Long-term follow-up studies are needed confirm this observation.

Among patients treated early in the disease course with antibiotics, the vast number do not develop chronic or serious complications. Unfortunately, there is a small fraction of early Lyme Disease patients who are treated and still develop chronic Lyme Disease. These are regarded as treatment failures.

In early Lyme Disease, diagnosis is generally made on the basis of two or more of the following: (1) living in an endemic Lyme region; (2) recollection of a tick bite; (3) presence of erythema migrans (EM); (4) exhibiting flu-like or constitutional symptoms. In the initial weeks of infection, blood tests may be negative because specific antibodies against the *Borrelia* spirochete are lacking. Generally, it requires 6 weeks to 3 months to develop a sufficiently high level of Lyme antibodies to test in the positive serum antibody range. In early localized Lyme Disease, waiting for the results of a blood test, which may be negative, can delay therapy and should be considered. Persons failing to meet several of the above criteria are difficult to diagnose. You and your physician should discuss potential risks of treating a disease you may not have. A physician's clinical experience with Lyme patients in endemic regions should also be considered.

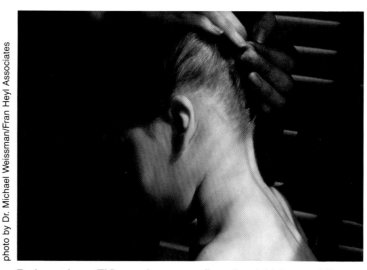

photo by Dr. Michael Weissman/Fran Heyl Associates

Erythema migrans (EM) appearing as a spreading redness behind young girl's ear.

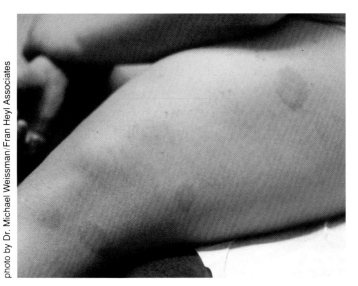

Secondary erythema migrans (EM) on a young boy's leg, appearing as multiple lesions once bacteria have spread in early disseminated Lyme disease.

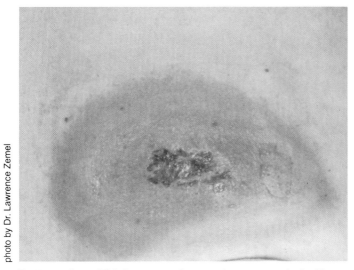

Erythema migrans (EM) that progressed to necrotic stage on man's shoulder.

LYME DISEASE
Clinical Signs & Symptoms

EARLY LOCALIZED STAGE
(days to weeks)

Erythema migrans (EM) appears as a classic reddish rash at the tick bite site, expanding outwardly from the center.

Swollen lymph nodes near the bite site are common.

Flu-like symptoms include headache, fever, chills, neck stiffness, aching muscles and joints, sore throat and fatigue.

EARLY DISSEMINATED STAGE
(weeks to months)

Aching muscles, tendons, and joints are common, usually in the knee or other large joint. Jaw pain is also reported.

Swollen lymph nodes at sites away from the bite site appear.

Secondary EM rash infrequently appears at remote sites, or a series of expanding, concentric rings sometimes develop.

Nervous system involvement includes severe headaches, facial palsy, muscle tics or twitching, balance problems, numbness or tingling in the extremities. Other complaints include lethargy, short-term memory loss, speech difficulties, disorientation, emotional instability, gait disturbances, or problems with sleep.

Heart problems present as irregular or skipped heartbeats, or temporary conduction blocks. Heart problems usually only last a few days to a week.

Problems with the eyes, ears, lungs, liver or stomach may occur. Some report instances of night sweats.

LATE DISSEMINATED STAGE
(months to years)

Chronic skin problems at the bite site occur rarely.

Prolonged, painful, swollen arthritic joints occur, often in the knees. Joint destruction can occur.

Chronic neurological problems include short-term memory loss, mental confusion, disorientation, intermittent paralysis and spasticity, and incapacitating fatigue.

Early Disseminated Lyme Disease

Within several weeks to months of the tick bite or appearance of EM, Lyme Disease enters the second phase. Dissemination means the spirochete has left the skin, appearing in other organs and tissues. Early disseminated Lyme Disease (Stage 2) may immediately follow early localized Lyme Disease. Or, the stages may be separated by one to three months, or even more. It is uncommon for the original EM to still be present at this stage. About 10% of patients do exhibit secondary EM at remote sites. Unlike the earliest manifestations of Lyme Disease, the clinical signs and symptoms are much more varied. Diagnosis at later stages is a challenge.

Migrating, intermittent joint pain lasting a few hours to a few days at a time is commonly seen. One or more joints may be affected during early disseminated Lyme Disease. The knee is the most frequently involved joint. Other large joints, such as the elbow, shoulder or pelvic girdles may be affected. Less frequently, the joints of the fingers, wrist, toes, or ankle become stiff and painful.

At this early stage, it is unusual to find joint swelling, warmth, and internal destruction of the joint. Occasionally, the temporomandibular joint (TMJ or jaw) is involved, accompanied by jaw-cracking and pain upon chewing. About one-third of patients will also experience pain in the thicker muscle belly, even when the muscle is at rest. Commonly, muscle pain (myalgia) is felt in one or more of the large muscles of the arm, hip, back, shoulder, or leg.

During early disseminated Lyme Disease, the spirochete may also invade the peripheral nerves, brain, and spinal cord. Estimates suggest nervous system involvement occurs in 15-30% of cases. Bacterial infection of the nervous system can produce meningitis, encephalitis, or even both. Meningitic signs and symptoms include severe headaches, dizziness and problems with balance, weakness or numbness in parts of the body, or tingling in the legs and/or arms. The numbness, weakness, or tingling may involve one or both extremities. One of the most commonly seen neurological signs is facial palsy, with loss of muscle tone on one side of the face. Often called Bell's palsy, a drooping eyelid and weakness in one corner of the mouth are common expressions of facial palsy.

Severe headaches may signal the onset of encephalitic signs, indicating brain inflammation. Other signs of encephalitis are much more subtle. These would include such complaints as sleep disturbances, inability to feel rested, difficulty in concentration, short-term memory losses, intermittent disorientation, and emotional instability. Only recently has the involvement of peripheral nerves been demonstrated. Due to nerve damage, measurable changes occur in the nerve impulse conduction speed. When Lyme Disease affects the peripheral nerves, loss of sensation, difficulty in gait, and fine tremors of the extremities may appear.

In addition to the joints, muscles, and nervous system, a small percentage (8-10%) of cases will experience difficulties with the heart. Disturbances in the impulse conduction system may produce some degree of heart block. In a few cases, the block has been severe enough to require a temporary pacemaker. Other cardiac symptoms include irregular heart beats and chest pains due to bacterial inflammation of the heart.

As experience with Lyme Disease grows, less frequent problems with sensory organs are being recognized. Bouts of conjunctivitis ("pink eye") cause the eye to burn, feel scratchy, or produce more mucous than usual. Blurred vision, narrowing of the visual fields (tunnel vision), sensations of pressure behind the eye, and eye pain have also been reported. When the inner ear or nerves supplying the ear are infected, hearing impairment, ringing in the ears, or sharp ear pain may result.

In most cases, by the time the signs of early disseminated Lyme disease begin appearing, antibodies directed against *Borrelia burgdorferi* are being produced and released to fight the infection. A serum blood test is often used to confirm a suspicion of Lyme disease. Again, remembrance of a tick bite or unusual skin rash, along with exposure to endemic areas, and consistent clinical signs and symptoms are invaluable in diagnosing Lyme Disease confidently.

Pregnancy and Lyme Disease

Borrelia burgdorferi during early localized Lyme Disease is carried in the bloodstream to other organs and tissues. This bacteria can also cross into the placental circulation and infect the fetus. But in mothers with chronic (late disseminated) Lyme Disease, few, if any, spirochetes remain in her circulation. So in late Lyme Disease, infection of the unborn is unlikely. Also, maternal anti-Lyme antibodies may help protect the unborn.

Care must be taken to avoid contracting Lyme Disease during pregnancy. The first trimester is the most critical time period because fetal organs are forming. In second and third trimesters, the formed organs are growing larger, starting to mature, becoming less susceptible to malformation. Fetal Lyme borreliosis has been suspected in some miscarriages, abnormalities, and developmental impairments, since spirochetes were cultured from fetal tissues. There are many reasons for miscarriages: one in five pregnancies miscarry. Further research is needed to understand the risk of Lyme Disease during pregnancy.

It now appears that the Lyme spirochete can be transmitted through the breast milk of infected mothers. Again, more work is needed to understand any potential risk to the infant. Should a pregnant woman contract Lyme Disease, effective antibiotics may be safely used under a physician's care. The antibiotic reaches both mother and fetus. At the onset of pregnancy, women living in Lyme endemic regions should discuss concerns about Lyme Disease with her obstetrician. Precautions might include the need to reduce or avoid risky behaviors (see **Preventive Measures Which Reduce Risk**).

photo by Dr. Michael Weissman/Fran Heyl Associates

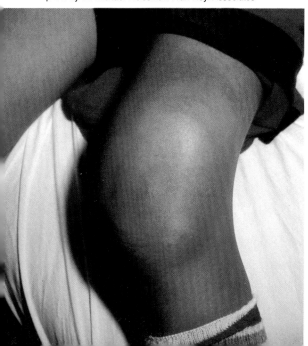

Arthritis in young boy's left knee due to late disseminated Lyme disease. Note characteristic joint swelling.

Late Disseminated Lyme Disease

Untreated patients may develop chronic Lyme Disease months to years later, frequently with long symptom-free intervals. Less is known about the manifestations of late disseminated Lyme Disease (Stage 3). Three reasons contribute: (1) the difficulty of diagnosis and the frequency of misdiagnosis; (2) the difficulty in conducting clinical trials in late Lyme patients where remissions can occur; and, (3) as with any "new" disease, knowledge is limited until research catches up with more answers.

About 10% of untreated patients can develop frank arthritis with swollen, painful, warm joints. Unlike earlier stages, the arthritis is not transient nor does it migrate from joint to joint. Much research is being directed at separating classic rheumatoid arthritis from late Lyme arthritis by using sophisticated serum tests for rheumatoid factor and other substances.

Analysis of the joint fluid (synovial fluid) and the joint itself has revealed the presence of only a few persistent spirochetes. In the late arthritic stage, there is erosive degeneration of the joint structure. And like rheumatoid arthritis, late Lyme arthritis may lead to severe impairments and permanent disability. With antibiotic therapy, reduction in pain and arrest of joint deterioration is expected in most of the patients with Lyme arthritis.

In perhaps 10-30% of late disseminated Lyme Disease patients, the nervous system is involved. The term "neuroborreliosis" describes neurological problems of late Lyme Disease. Included in this profile are short-term memory loss, mental confusion and disorientation, a rolling, stumbling gait, cognitive disturbances, especially in abstract thinking and problem solving, partial spastic paralysis, and even dementia. The fatigue accompanying late disseminated Lyme Disease is described as severe, unrelenting, incapacitating, extreme, and unremitting.

Because it is so varied, it is not surprising that neuroborreliosis has been misdiagnosed. It has been mistaken for multiple sclerosis (MS), amyotrophic lateral sclerosis (ALS or Lou Gehrig's disease), lupus, herpes encephalitis, chronic fatigue syndrome, brain tumor, psychiatric disorders, and even

Alzheimer's disease. Of course, none of these conditions would receive antibiotic therapy. Late nervous system Lyme Disease has been called the great imitator because it resembles so many other diseases. Intensive research is directed at several tests which will distinguish Lyme neuroborreliosis from other nervous system disorders. *Borreliae* persist in the nervous tissue and are somewhat protected from the general circulation. As such, patience and prolonged therapy are needed to reduce or control neurological Lyme infections. Some healing and a gradual return of function is expected over time in all but the most severe cases.

Diagnosis of Lyme Disease

Diagnosis is the art and the science of identifying a disease from its signs and symptoms. Of all the signs and symptoms relating to Lyme Disease, erythema migrans (EM) is considered the classical hallmark sign of early localized Lyme Disease. Its early appearance may resemble a bacterial infection of the skin or a reaction to a spider bite. But the expansion of the red ring and typical central clearing with time suggests Lyme Disease with a high degree of certainty. If EM is accompanied by several constitutional symptoms, if the person lives in an endemic area, and if a tick bite at the site can be recalled, a confident diagnosis of Lyme Disease is made. In persons lacking a classical EM or having an atypical rash, diagnostic certainty is lowered.

Several weeks to months later, diagnosis of early disseminated Lyme Disease is more difficult when there is a wider variety of signs and symptoms. Most infected patients will show elevated serum antibodies against *Borreliae* within 6 weeks to 3 months. But a small percentage convert from negative to positive antibody levels (seroconversion) at longer intervals. Thus, diagnosis on the basis of serum antibodies **alone** is insufficient for a confident diagnosis of Lyme Disease. Patient history and clinical examination are just as important to the physician.

Uncommonly, some individuals do not develop an immune response against the spirochete. If no antibodies are made, there is nothing to detect. Several reasons for the lack of an immune response have been offered: (1) antibiotics given for other problems removed the bacteria (immune stimulus) before an antibody response could be launched; (2) use of drugs with immunosuppressive properties (steroids, anti-inflammatory drugs) may have blunted the immune reaction so that few antibodies are present; and (3) the Lyme bacteria may have disappeared quickly from the circulation into other tissues before immune defenses reacted.

Clinical data support the first two reasons, and laboratory animal studies support the latter reason. In some cases of late disseminated Lyme Disease involving the nervous system (neuroborreliosis), clinicians have observed the presence of Lyme antibodies in the cerebrospinal fluid (CSF) obtained by spinal tap when Lyme antibodies are absent or too low to detect in the serum.

Two types of diagnostic tests are commonly used for detecting high levels of Lyme antibodies in the serum or CSF. These tests do not prove or disprove that a patient has Lyme Disease. Instead the tests identify antibodies, but not the actual bacteria causing Lyme Disease. Immunofluorescence assays (IFA) react serum antibodies against the spirochete using laboratory-prepared mixtures of Lyme antigens. The fluorescence from the antigen-antibody binding is observed under a fluorescence microscope. Enzyme-linked immunosorbent assays (ELISA) also react Lyme antigens with serum anti-Lyme antibodies. Reaction with a specific enzyme produces a color change, similar to over-the-counter pregnancy tests.

Laboratories are actively working on many fronts to improve diagnostic assay quality. The questions being addressed by researchers are many. Which bacterial antigens of *Borrelia burgdorferi* do most humans produce antibodies against (diagnostic sensitivity)? Are the antigens specific only for *Borrelia burgdorferi*, or will other spirochetes or even other bacteria also cause the same or similar antibodies to be produced (diagnostic specificity)? What group of individuals (blood donors?) are the best controls? Do "healthy" residents lack specific Lyme antibodies or cross-reacting antibodies (i.e., syphilis)? Is there a way to identify the antigen itself, instead of antibodies against the antigen?

All diagnostic assays attempt to achieve a delicate balance of high sensitivity without sacrificing specificity for the disease in question. If sensitivity is high, some false positive outcomes may result when a lower specificity is introduced. A false positive result identifies a person as having Lyme Disease when they really don't. A lower sensitivity accompanied by a higher

LYME DISEASE
SURVEILLANCE CRITERIA

Prior to January 1, 1991, each state reported cases of Lyme Disease within that state according to each state's case definition. Counting by defined criteria allowed each state health department to assess whether Lyme Disease was a growing problem, or was it moving into new areas, or was it decreasing. An epidemiologic case definition is intended for surveillance (counting) purposes **ONLY**.

States using a broader definition would be expected to count more cases of Lyme Disease than those states using a more strict, narrower case definition. Beginning in 1991, the US Centers for Disease Control enacted a uniform case definition for Lyme Disease on a nationwide basis, superceding each state's own definition. Physicians are mandated by law to report new cases of Lyme Disease to local health departments.

CDC CASE DEFINITION –
SURVEILLANCE CRITERIA – 1991

A case of Lyme Disease is defined as follows:

1. A person with erythema migrans (EM); **OR**
2. A person with laboratory confirmation of infection **AND** at least one late manifestation:
   a. Involvement of the musculoskeletal system (recurrent, brief attacks of joint swelling in one or a few joints)
   b. Involvement of the nervous system (lymphocytic meningitis, cranial neuritis, especially facial palsy, radiculoneuropathy, or rarely, encephalomyelitis)
   c. Involvement of the cardiovascular system (acute onset of high grade AV conduction block which resolves in days to weeks, and possibly myocarditis)

MINNESOTA CASE DEFINITION PRIOR TO 1991:

1. A person with erythema migrans (EM) witnessed by a physician.

WISCONSIN CASE DEFINITION PRIOR TO 1991:

1. A person with erythema migrans (EM) following exposure to an endemic region occurring no more than 30 days earlier; **OR**
2. A person without EM that has involvement of at least one of three organ systems (as above)
   AND
   a. a positive serologic test for Lyme Disease
   OR
   b. isolation of *Borrelia burgdorferi* from a clinical specimen.

specificity will produce more false negative results. A false negative result misses people who do have Lyme Disease. **Ideally,** there should be no false positive or negative test results. Nearly all of the commercially-available diagnostic tests are good, helping a physician diagnose Lyme Disease. But there is still room to improve both sensitivity and specificity.

Diagnosis of Lyme Disease represents a medical challenge, to be sure. But the use of demographic data (endemic exposure), recollection of a tick bite, presence of EM, a positive serum and/or CSF test, and the involvement of one or more organ systems consistent with Lyme Disease must all be carefully weighed. Finally, a good therapeutic response to antibiotic drugs active against spirochetes suggests that some kind of bacterial infection was present, but it may or may not have been Lyme Disease.

Treatment of Lyme Disease

During early localized Lyme Disease while the EM is still present, the treatment of choice is a 2-3 week course of oral antibiotics. Which antibiotic is selected is based upon the patient's age, history, possible allergies, and physician's experiences with Lyme Disease. Most often, the oral antibiotic is chosen from the penicillin, tetracycline or cephalosporin classes. Very few patients develop secondary Lyme symptoms following antibiotic treatment for early disease. From the work done to date, immunity to Lyme Disease does not appear to develop and reinfection is possible.

In-dwelling catheter for infusion of intravenous antibiotic drug for treatment of late disseminated Lyme Disease.

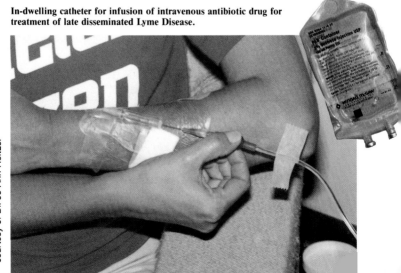

During early and late disseminated stages of Lyme Disease, the physician can choose between the intravenous route and the oral routes. Length of treatment as well as the need for retreatment or combination-antibiotic regimens are decisions made by the physician based upon the patient's response to therapy, the patient's history, and the newest advances being made in Lyme Disease therapy.

One of the most difficult areas of therapeutic research is the conduct of controlled clinical trials. In chronic long-term Lyme Disease it is often difficult to diagnose and evaluate patient improvement. While currently-used therapies are successful in most patients, several different approaches may have to be tried in one individual. Clinical data are lacking that allow us to estimate what percentage of late stage Lyme patients achieve cures or long-lasting remissions.

Risks of Contracting Lyme Disease

The reason one gets Lyme Disease, quite simply put, is because an infected tick bit and fed for a day or more. Thus, any behaviors which reduce the likelihood of either human-to-tick contact or the length of tick feeding must be considered risk-reducing, if not totally preventive. Knowing which areas may be infested with a high proportion of infected ticks is not always possible. Precautions should always be taken. Being in contact with vegetation where field mice, deer, rabbits, racoons, or ground-feeding birds are, or where freely-roaming pets may have transported infected ticks, constitutes a risk. Even small lizards transport infected ticks in parts of California.

Several years ago it was felt that fields of tall grass bordering woodlands and marshes were the only spots where humans got Lyme Disease. Today, the disease has moved into suburban neighborhoods, including mown lawns, and even city parks in some endemic areas, where deer are infrequently seen.

Some information on tick infestation of neighborhoods or parks is available from some local county and state health departments. Each agency is now involved in nationwide surveillance for Lyme Disease. Universities and wildlife resource management agencies also collect data on spirochetal infection rates of ticks within some locales. Occasionally, newspapers may report infectivity rates (what % of ticks carry *Borreliae*) and infestation rates (how many ticks are there) prior to scientific publication.

Risk is first and foremost associated with the abundance of *Ixodes dammini* in proximity to potential human hosts. Studies show that the abundance of deer in an area correlates to the abundance of *Ixodes* ticks. Near eradication of deer in controlled locales has markedly reduced tick density. To a large degree, the risk of getting Lyme Disease is also related to the availability of other suitable hosts (rabbit, mice, raccoon, etc.), the ranging behavior of infected hosts (birds, deer, dog), and favorable climate, habitat, and geography.

Make the home and yard a less desirable environment for ticks, mice, and deer. Remove brush and weedy areas near the house. Move birdfeeders away from the house since mice are attracted to the dropped seeds. Do not encourage deer to come into the yard by feeding them. Consider using safe pesticides in the carpet and pet bedding. One ingenius patented product, using acaricide-treated (kills ticks) cotton balls, may result in fewer tick-infested mice in the yard. This product may not be practical for homeowners due to a limited duration of effect, giving a false sense of security, and its high cost.

The second half of the risk equation relates to human behavior. **Unlike** syphilis or AIDS which is transmitted through sexual behaviors and/or infected blood contact, Lyme Disease is far easier to contract through routine behaviors common to a large segment of society. Human contact with an infected tick can occur during hiking and hunting, during yard work and gardening, or during outdoor play and recreation. Or it may occur by transfer of an unattached, infected tick from house pets allowed to roam in infested areas. Two recent studies evaluating human risk factors have shown positive correlations with lawn mowing and, to a lesser extent, with pet ownership. Children, owing to the amount of time they spend outdoors, typically are at greater risk than most adults.

According to laboratory animal studies, once bitten by an infected tick, it is believed that at least 12-24 hours of feeding are needed before the spirochetal infection passes to the host's bloodstream. Typically, a feeding tick will remain attached to the host for 3-5 days and then drop off. The 12-24 hour safety margin provides adequate time to search for and remove attached or crawling ticks (body checks). **More than any other habit, frequent and thorough body checks will significantly reduce your risk of getting Lyme Disease.** It may be difficult, if not impossible, to reduce many risk behaviors substantially, or impact the interactions of the bacteria, the tick, and the host animal, but preventive behaviors (outlined below), adopted as habits, can markedly reduce your risk of contracting Lyme Disease.

Preventive Measures Which Reduce Risk

Reducing the chance of human-to-tick contact is at the root of all preventive measures. Even among the 8 endemic states, tick infectivity rates vary from virtually none to 70% or more. Not only is the tick population growing successfully, host infectivity is also increasing within these populations. This favors the spread of human and veterinary Lyme Disease. Studies show that tick habitat and the host animals carrying ticks are expanding from woodlands and wildlife preserves into ever closer contact with human environs - the places where we live, play, and work. Therefore, knowing that the tick is out there is the first step in reducing risk.

Clothing can be a formidable deterrent for ticks. Hungry larval ticks remain close to the ground, generally feeding on field mice and other small animals. Nymphal and adult ticks crawl upward to the tips of vegetation (questing behavior) seeking contact with a warm-blooded host. Whenever possible, wear long pants tucked into the socks, boots or socks pulled over the calf. Ticks climb upward so that the first contact with human flesh can be controlled by how the clothing are worn. Shirts tucked in at the waist encourage the tick to continue its upward climb in search of skin contact. Wearing long-sleeved shirts or cuffed apparel may also help.

Frequent vigorous brushing of the clothing with the hand can help dispel climbing ticks. Wearing light-colored clothing makes it easier to spot climbing ticks and remove them. In a recent newsletter of the Bluebird Restoration Association of Wisconsin, a patented outerwear garment called Tick Chaps™ was described. This innovative idea uses a midthigh tick flap (an inverted pleat) to delay upward crawling of the tick. By adding an insect repellent to the inner aspect of the flap, your chances of tick contact with open skin are markedly reduced.

In addition to wearing clothing which discourages tick attachment, there can be no substitute for thorough body checks after being outdoors or in contact with outdoor animals. Nymphal and adult ticks are exceedingly small. Careful examination of the body, including skin folds, ears, navel, and scalp is necessary. Whenever possible, after being outdoors, vigorously scrub the skin with a wrung-out wash cloth. This helps dislodge any crawling ticks which might have escaped notice. An attached tick should be carefully removed (see page 29).

The routine use of insect repellents cannot be encouraged unless absolutely necessary. Read the manufacturer's warning: children are **MORE** sensitive than adults to repellents, such as DEET. If you must be in tick-infested brush or fields, use repellents intended for the skin with caution (see warning label). These repellents can also provide a false sense of invulnerability. Tick or insect repellents that are designed for application to clothing (not skin) may be applied to boots, shoes, socks, pants, and sleeves.

PREVENTING LYME DISEASE
BY REDUCING RISK

- AVOID TICK INFESTED AREAS

- WEAR SENSIBLE, PROTECTIVE CLOTHING
  - Tuck pants into socks
  - Select light-colored clothing
  - Brush clothing often
  - Use repellents carefully

- PERFORM FREQUENT BODY CHECKS
  - Check skin folds, scalp & neck
  - Scrub with damp cloth

- MAKE HOME LESS DESIRABLE HABITAT
  - Remove brush and weedy areas
  - Move birdfeeders away from home
  - Discourage deer in lawn
  - Consider pesticides in carpet, pet bedding

- PROTECT YOUR PETS
  - Perform coat and body checks
  - Use tick collars, sprays, powders (check with veterinarian)

- KEEP A HEALTH JOURNAL OR CALENDAR
  - Note insect bites, rashes
  - Note travel to endemic areas
  - Record flu-like episodes

Manufacturers' claims indicate that products containing 30% DEET or 0.5% permethrin (sold as Permanone) are nearly 100% effective in repelling deer ticks. The ability of these repellent products to kill deer ticks is far less. Sealing outdoor clothing into plastic bags until laundered may be necessary to prevent the home from becoming infested. Pets and other large animals may carry infected ticks to persons, their yards, and their homes so that some precautions are warranted (see below).

Because the EM rash is not always present and the signs and symptoms of early localized Lyme Disease are quite general and nondescript, keeping a health journal on yourself, your family, and pets is a good idea. Use a family calendar to note suspicious insect bites, unusual outdoor activities, travel to endemic locales, and bouts with flu-like episodes. Include the dates and duration of problems. Your physician will find these records useful if you begin to suspect Lyme Disease.

If you already suspect that you may have contracted Lyme Disease, begin to chart problems you consider unusual (severe headaches, slurred speech, stiff neck, etc.). Be creative in defining your "problem" in a measurable way, such as time of day, length of activity before fatigue sets in, situations which generated atypical or inconsistent behavior, etc. For a physician, your objective records are invaluable tools for making a diagnosis and monitoring therapeutic progress.

Veterinary Lyme Disease

House pets, if allowed outdoors, may serve as inadvertent transporters of infected ticks into the home. After checking with your veterinarian, tick collars, sprays, and powders may be suggested. The veterinarian is quite likely to understand the local risk of contracting Lyme Disease since outdoor animals generally acquire the illness earlier than their owners. If you live in an area where conditional animal vaccines are available, be aware that vaccinated animals may still serve as transporters of the tick. Body checks of indoor-outdoor pets should be routinely performed, looking carefully around the eyes, ears, mouth, groin, and "armpits" of the pet. Check the coat for crawling ticks. Use of fine-toothed combs and bathing pets may remove crawling ticks, but attached ticks will remain, posing a risk to the pet. On short-haired dogs or cats, tape-type lint removers may be used to remove crawling ticks.

According to the most recent estimates, Lyme Disease appears to be six times more common in outdoor dogs than their owners. It is unclear whether these dogs collect that many more ticks, spend that much more time outdoors, or have an increased susceptibility to Lyme Disease, or some combination of these factors. In the dog, the earliest signs of Lyme Disease usually involve lameness or soreness in the hip or neck. Abrupt changes in the dog's normal behavior, such as no longer jumping on the sofa or failing to walk stairs, can be an early sign. Erythema migrans, however, can be spotted by careful examination of the pet by an informed owner. Cats, on the other hand, more often exhibit signs of nervous system involvement, again, rather abruptly. For example, jumping to a chair and appearing clumsy and uncoordinated. Cats, by virtue of their incessant grooming, tend to be at lower risk than dogs.

Lyme Disease can also affect large farm animals such as cattle, sheep, and horses. In these animals, arthritis which comes and goes is usually the first sign of Lyme Disease. If untreated, it progresses to classic arthritis with permanent impairment. As in humans, Lyme Disease diagnostic tests are useful when paired with other information. The early illness in animals usually responds very well to antibiotic management.

Check your pet carefully for crawling or attached deer ticks. Remove tick with caution.

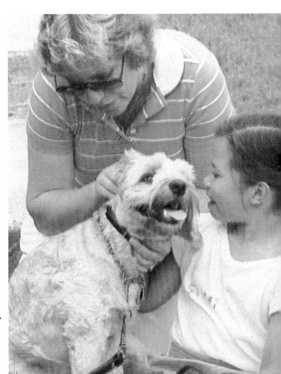

courtesy of Pfizer Central Research

Removing an Attached Tick

If an attached tick is found, it is likely to have burrowed its head into the skin. Extreme care must be used. **DO NOT GRASP THE BODY OF THE TICK!** Using a fine tweezers, grasp the tick as close to the head as possible and gently pull until the tick loosens its grip. Often flesh will be attached to the tick. If you squeeze the body of an infected tick, the midgut contents could be expelled directly into the bloodstream, greatly increasing your chances of contracting Lyme Disease. After the tick has been removed, aggressively wash the bite site with soap and warm water, followed by rubbing alcohol or hydrogen peroxide. Continue to watch the bite site for one month for signs of EM. If a rash appears, see your physician immediately.

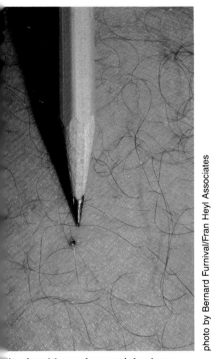

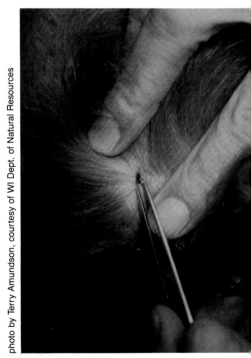

photo by Bernard Furnival/Fran Heyl Associates

photo by Terry Amundson, courtesy of WI Dept. of Natural Resources

...ing deer tick nymph on man's leg shown
   pencil point. Remove feeding ticks
...fully.

Remove attached deer tick carefully with a fine tweezers. Grasping as close to the skin as possible, pull gently until tick loosens its grip. Do NOT squeeze tick.

If the tick is being saved for later identification, place it in an inverted jar with a tight- fitting cap and a moistened cotton ball. The tick can remain alive for several weeks. Recall that the tick will attempt to crawl upward, so that inverting the jar is a prudent measure. If there is no need to save the tick, the best way to dispose of it is to impale the tick on a pin and burn the tick with a match. Dead ticks may be preserved in rubbing alcohol to teach others about Lyme Disease.

Impact of Lyme Disease

If Lyme Disease progresses to a chronic condition, the cost to the patient in terms of health, dollars, career, and interpersonal relationships can be enormous. Misdiagnosis and inappropriate treatment only add to these costs. Diminished productivity and lowered self-esteem are unavoidable consequences of untreated late stage Lyme Disease. Measures you and your family can employ will markedly lower your risk of contracting Lyme Disease.

For a few, it may be too late to avoid chronic Lyme Disease, but there is much which can be done for all phases of the disease if medical attention is sought promptly. As with any "new" disease, active research continues expanding our knowledge of Lyme Disease, evaluating better diagnostics and treatment protocols, and testing different means of controlling environmental factors to decrease the spread of Lyme Disease.

For the foreseeable future, Lyme Disease is here to stay in Minnesota and Wisconsin, and it may reach endemic proportions in other surrounding states. This reference booklet has been written with the intent of providing enough information about Lyme Disease and its consequences so that you can make responsible decisions about protecting yourself and your family. With this reference booklet, the information is in one place, helping you understand how Lyme Disease is spread, what behaviors reduce your risk, and when you should seek medical attention quickly.

GLOSSARY

ACARICIDE   (ah·**CARE**·eh·side)
A substance with tick-killing properties

ANTIBIOTIC   (**AN**·ti·bi·**OT**·ick)
Class of prescription drug which is used to slow or halt bacterial growth

ANTIBODY   (**AN**·ti·**BOD**·ee)
Substance made by the body to neutralize or destroy bacteria, viruses, or toxins

ANTIGEN   (**AN**·tah·gen)
Any substance such as a bacteria that causes the body to produce antibodies; something which looks foreign to the body

BORRELIA BURGDORFERI (bor·**REEL**·ee·ah burg·**DOOR**·fur·ee)
The Latin name of the bacteria which infects the host and causes Lyme Disease; it is carried by ticks

CARDIAC   (**KAR**·dee·ack)
Pertaining to the heart or heart linings

CHRONIC   (**KRON**·ick)
Medically, lasting a long time or marked by frequent recurrences, generally for longer than 6 months

CONSTITUTIONAL   (kon·sta·**TOO**·shun·al)
Affecting the physical makeup or well-being of the body, such as flu-like symptoms of achiness or nausea

DISSEMINATED (dis·**SEM**·in·ay·ted)
Spreading to two or more organs or tissues in the body

ENDEMIC   (en·**DEM**·ick)
Continuing on a widespread basis; a disease which is always expected to be present in a locale

ERYTHEMA MIGRANS   (air·ah·**THEEM**·ah **MY**·grans)
Typical skin rash around a tick bite site in early Lyme Disease, usually appears as an enlarging redness with a clear center

HOST
An animal which feeds a parasite (tick), usually by providing blood

IMMUNE RESPONSE (im·**YOON** ree·**SPONS**)
Producing antibodies to defend against an invading bacteria or other type of antigen

IXODES DAMMINI   (ix·**O**·dees **DAM**·in·eye)
The Latin name for the deer tick; Ixodes refers to a classification of small, hard-bodied ticks

NEUROLOGICAL   (noor·oh·**LODGE**·ick·all)
Pertaining to the nerves, brain, or spinal cord

RELAPSE (**REE**·laps)
Return of symptoms after a period of time

REMISSION (ree·**MISH**·un)
Disappearance of symptoms for a period of time

SERUM (**Seer**·um)
Portion of blood remaining after cells and clotting factors are removed; portion of blood containing antibodies

SIGNS
Tests which a doctor uses to measure function, such as a knee-jerk reflex or reduced range-of-motion

SPIROCHETE (**SPY**·roh·keet)
Classification of coiled, corkscrew-shaped bacteria; typically slow-growing and persistent

SYMPTOMS (**SIM**·tums)
Complaints made by a patient that cannot be seen or measured, such as fatigue or soreness

TREPONEMA PALLIDUM (trep·o·**KNEE**·ma **PAL**·lid·um)
Latin name for the spirochete which causes syphilis

VECTOR (**VECK**·tor)
A carrier, such as a tick, which transmits bacteria to its host; a line of transmission

Tick Chaps is a trademark owned by Carl McIlquham.

"Permanone" is permethrin, manufactured by Fairfield American of Newark, NJ, and marketed solely by Coulston International of Easton, PA.

"DEET" is diethyltoluamide, a chemical marketed as an insect repellent by several manufacturers.